Tea, Tips & Tricks

ALSO BY BIODUN ABUDU

Tales of My Skin

Stolen Sanity

Forbidden Scriptures

Open Letters From Within

Tea, Tips & Tricks

Biodun Abudu

www.BiodunAbudu.com

ISBN-13: 978-1-7335910-5-8

This is a book that shares knowledge that I have acquired through my journey. I am not a health professional or expert but I do provide information to the best of my knowledge. Certain tips and tricks are to be used at your own risk. For the tea (tea means juicy gossip) portion it's usually verified tea that was delivered to my doorstep. Hope you enjoy and find the information in this book helpful!

Table of Contents

Cleaning

Cleaning Tips 101

Here are a few cleaning tips and tricks that are already known to some of us, but are still not common for others. These cleaning tips are amazing and very easy!

a.   **Vinegar** - Cleaning your mirror with vinegar and water is the most amazing thing ever. It is perfect for avoiding those mirror streaks when cleaning. Mix the right amount of vinegar and water in a spray bottle. Spray the solution and clean with a cloth.

b. **Lemon** - Cleaning your microwave with lemon is amazing. Slice the lemon in half, squeeze the juice into the bowl with water then throw the halves in.

Microwave on high power for about 3 minutes. Leave in there for about 5 minutes and then wipe with a clean cloth. For the tougher stains, just dip the cloth in the lemon water and scrub until it's removed.

c. **Mr. Clean** - So we all have those moments when we are super pissed looking at the crayon stains left on your white walls by kids or even random permanent marks left by adults during a house party. The annoying one is when you have visitors who somehow scratch your walls with their luggage. Well, I have a simple solution to remove those stains. Mr. Clean magic eraser (white colored sponge) is perfect on white walls that have been stained with permanent markers or any other kind of stains.

Wet the tip or part of the Mr. Clean magic eraser with water and proceed to gently wipe off that permanent marker on the white wall. After wiping away gently with no visible traces, you can leave the wall to dry off on its own. It will be like it was never there, I tell you. This is much easier than going to buy paint for a little mark made by kids or by friends who are visiting your home and use their luggage to scratch your walls.

Electronic & Internet

Zero Worries

Home Cameras - These are very beneficial to everyone for peace of mind and security. Home security cameras are not only for home owners, but also for people who stay in apartments (even in studio apartments). Especially apartment buildings where the maintenance team in your building owns a master key to unlock everyone's door, this is helpful. This also would be good even for those who rent a room with five other people. You can find affordable security cameras that require wifi and an outlet for power. These little cameras use memory cards allowing a large memory space. They alert you and immediately start recording when they detect movement in your room or apartment. You can talk into the camera as well and also listen to sounds.

This would be helpful when you're at work and are worried about what the maintenance team is doing while they are fixing your refrigerator or sink. This also helps to know if your new roommate is going into your bedroom without your consent. You can zoom in on images or faces in the video, you can download the video to watch on your computer and more. Hopefully you never will need to download videos to show the police and zoom in on the person's face, but it's comforting to know the camera is there if needed.

Lastly, this camera would also be great for when someone has a new home health aide or nurse that comes to check on our autistic child or grandparents. This also works for mothers with newborns who are leaving their child with a new babysitter.

God forbid there is any form of abuse, but if there is, you can catch it on camera. This seems like something we would all know, but not everyone thinks of having a little security camera at home that they can place in a hidden corner. Some of us have gotten too comfortable calling a million times with FaceTime to ask our child if he or she is okay thinking the child will always speak through FaceTime. Speeding through traffic to get home and open the door randomly won't help that much either.

A camera will definitely give you a replay option to see what happened all through the day for your peace of mind.

Searching Deep

We at times may come across images that we need to find their original roots. We stumble across pictures and we need to get more info on the creator. I have used Yandex for reverse image searching and it provides the exact pic from its original root (whether on facebook or a particular website) and also provides similar images as well.

Yandex only shows where the image is being used; if the image is not found, it usually shows similar images. This also helps to provide other pictures of the person you are searching for or even provide images of the person on websites their pictures have been featured on. Yandex provide links below the image so you can go directly to the website where the image is featured. It is a strong search engine for face matching and location identification besides Google image search.

Facebook Networking

I never knew how useful Facebook groups really were till I desperately needed help and I joined one. On Facebook you can search for many kinds of topics/things (for example: art, sports, food, teachers, hairstylists, etc.) you're interested in and request to join the groups. In these groups you can find people with different levels of experience. You can post questions and anyone will answer them. For example you can ask a question like, "Can anyone advise me on what manufacturing companies are the best for creating wigs?" Then people in the group will answer and may even share their experiences with the companies.

You can even find people advertising their events in these groups. Anyone can attend these events and network with like minded individuals that may share tips on ways you can elevate within the industry. I have seen times where magazines join these groups and ask the members in there if anyone would like to be featured in their next issue. It's very possible for you to join a music artists' group on facebook and someone could share an opportunity in the group with others for a potential opportunity to sign with a huge music label. You just never know what vital information you can stumble across in there. These Facebooks groups are very useful and often overlooked. Keep in mind that these facebook groups have rules, and I advise going over them before posting anything.

Google Helper

Have you ever felt like you needed to get the name of a store but really don't have any idea what it might be? You also don't even know the address of the store and neither do any of your friends or family. Here is a tip to finding the name and address of the store.

You will need to use the street view on Google Maps on your cellular phone. To do this, all you have to do is open the Google Maps app on your phone. Then, click on the search bar and enter the name or address of the place you can remember which is closest to the store you have forgotten. After this, click the small photo box on the left side (usually lower part) of the screen; it will have the 360 sign on it.

Once you click on it, it will have a street view and on the top will be a copyright sign with 2021 Google written there. To find the name or address of the store you need, or are looking for, just move the screen along the blue lines showing on the street (using your memory to navigate) until you reach the area of where the store is. When you reach an identifiable area, zoom in and write down the store name and address. From there, just search Google using their name or address and get their number and store hours.

Specific Fonts

If you are ever searching for a particular font you saw online and want to use it, you can check on WhatFontIs.com. You can easily upload the image of the font you are searching for and the website will give you results on where you can download the font for free or possibly purchase it.

Power of Hashtags

A lot of people don't realize the power of hashtags when it comes to building your brand or business online. You can find so many opportunities, networking events, potential buyers and more. When you search for certain hashtags, you can stumble across many people that are interested in what you have to offer. For example, let's say you are a wine maker and you need to find customers or stores to place your wine in. You can search #WineLover and #WineStore on Instagram, Twitter etc. When you search for those hashtags it will bring up millions of people's profiles who have used one of these hashtags under their pictures. When you click on the person's profile you can then dm(direct message) them or email them about your brand. If you searched #WineStore, you can click on search results and click on profiles and send proposals to wine stores you come across to market your product. You can scroll through the store's profile to see what they are about, how they respond to customers, when last they posted and more before emailing them to collaborate with them. Even when you post you can use certain hashtags and potential customers can even find you from them searching those particular hashtags also.

If you are visiting another city and want to see what you can attend, you can search #NewYorkEvents and scroll through pictures to see recent posts that have events in the month or week you are visiting. Sometimes you can stumble across dance auditions if you are a dancer looking to get into the industry. You can just search #DanceCompanies or #DanceAuditions or #Dancers (to see what other dancers are up to so you can also be a part of it).

Tech Tip

This is a tip a friend shared with me online. If you mistakenly close a word document without saving it and there was no autosave for it, what you can do is open the "My/This PC" in your file explorer and type ".asd". You'll find the document there.

The ASD file was created by Microsoft Word as a temporary backup. It is mostly known to be used for automatically generated backups.

Scrolling Through iPhone Text Msgs

This tip is to show you how to find certain information in your iPhone messages instead of scrolling over super lengthy text conversations, especially if you and the person talk almost everyday.

 What I usually do is think of a word I used in that particular month or period with that person. Then you can search that particular word in the iPhone text message search bar. It will then show all your text conversations with the word you searched. Scroll down after this and select which text looks familiar around that period with the person you had the conversation with, of course. Click on the text message and scroll to find what you are looking for. This saves time rather than scrolling through 6 months worth of conversations.

For example, a friend of mine was looking for the price of the items her husband had bought for their son's party. She knew the text message she was looking for was around October, but she felt overwhelmed scrolling all the way to October 2020 from February 2021. I told her to think of a word that will help her locate the conversation easier. She remembered the word "Lion King" which was the theme of the party she did for her son around that period. She searched "Lion King" in the iPhone text message search bar and scrolled down to click on the conversation she recognized in October of the year 2020. From that point in the text message, it wasn't hard to scroll to find exactly what she needed.

Protect Your Privacy

Some of us want to share our vacation trips, but not necessarily give everything away while we are on the trip. This is because we still want to show off a little, but still stay protected. I once saw in a movie that people keep tabs on you and when they know you are on vacation, they come rob your house unless you have someone who's at home still. I am a firm believer of uploading vacation photos after a trip. It's also fun to upload photos without the location (keep those girls or your ex guessing).

While you are on the trip, if you must upload, you can upload food pics and certain backgrounds with no location.

Proper Social Media Break

I understand that we all need a mental break from social media, especially from the negativity it sometimes has on there. I do have to say stop deleting or deactivating your Instagram page! If you are a business owner and or a creator and you need a break from social media, just delete the app without deleting or deactivating your profile. It upsets me to look for someone on social media and I come across a blank profile with the "no posts yet" written on their profile or the "user not found" written on their profile. I have no way to get their email, phone number or to see their created work or products. You are supposed to leave your page the way it is and just temporarily delete the app so potential clients can still DM you for work or with questions. Upon your return after you redownload the app, you can then go through your messages for potential work.

Health

Ashy

So, if you don't know, some of us have ashy feet and we are made fun of when noticed. So, to avoid these moments I'll be providing a few techniques to hide your ashy feet. Solutions are key, but I want to provide what you need if you are outside and can't run to exfoliate your legs at the moment.

a. **Covered Shoes** - Have full covered shoes like toms that can fit in your bag. This saves you from embarrassment during summer after you have walked a long period of time in sandals which don't cover your ashy feet.

b. **Oils** - Take foot oils that come in travel-sizes that you can rub on your feet the moment you notice their getting ashy or are ashy. With the oil you can mix in a pinch of sunscreen to protect your feet especially if you are wearing sandals or flip flops.

c. **Exfoliating** - Regular exfoliating solutions can help over time. You can soak your feet in warm water and use a pumice stone to eliminate the flakes and get other dead skin off your feet. Use the best soaps to wash. Then use the best moisturizers and oils to rub your feet, wearing socks that aid in locking in moisture overnight. Doing this will help in reducing dry feet also known as ashy feet.

Hide That Belly

Chile! So when I moved into my building I literally had only been to the gym the one time the leasing officer was showing me around the building. The other time I attempted to go in there was just to take a selfie. In fact, I tried again to go there to see someone cute working out, lol. But seriously, generally, some of us need several ways to hide our belly. Not all of us are familiar with the gym or pushing themselves to the point of almost passing out while doing pushups. Some of us (including myself) can't even spell gym, unfortunately, lol. However, we have temporary solutions to hide our bellies till we are mentally ready to work out.

a. **Corset** - Corsets help to flatten and to cover our belly fat temporarily though. These shouldn't be worn to sleep because it cuts off circulation and makes it difficult to breathe. (This can also be a waist trainer instead of a corset).

b. **Black** - Wearing black clothing really does help to hide our belly fat depending on the style of the black clothing you are wearing.

c. **Suck It** - The good ole "Suck it in" for the photos helps also. However, don't forget to smile during the photos or else you will look constipated.

d. **No Stripes** – Don't wear horizontal stripes as it makes you look bigger.

e. **Angles** - Knowing your angles when taking photos can also make you look slimmer, and for the women getting their picture taken, curvier.

MotherLand Tip

a.   **Water and Soap** - Water and soap can be used to wash up after a bowel movement. It might be a foreign idea to a lot of people, but some of us are already used to this in other countries. It's actually the safest way to clean up. Using tissue paper actually can be harsh to the private area's delicate skin. A lot of people don't know this and it's no wonder why people went crazy during the 2020 covid pandemic over tissue in the stores. Wet wipes are of course way better than tissue and clean better.

However, I don't expect people to carry water and soap to public spaces, so wet wipes would be a better option than tissue. If you're at home, then save your coins and use water and soap. Water is environmentally friendly also.

No Visible Spots

Hidden Hair Chronicles - Not everyone can afford hair transplant surgeries which can cost from $4,000 to $15,000. I'm not even talking about monthly payments for a tv advertised hair solution that could cost over $200 per month. Well, here are a few things you can do temporarily to hide that bald spot or thin hair.

a.   **Hair Fibers** - Hair fibers work miracles and it's what most people use on a movie set in Hollywood. The hair fibers (Toppik, Regain) are fabulous either in a fiber powder form or a spray. The hair fibers after a few minutes blend in with your regular hair and cover that bald shiny spot on your head. When you use the hair fiber, you are to avoid swimming and the rain because it will spill your tea and wash all of it out causing a scene wherever you are. For extra protection, you can use hair grease lightly and pour the hair fiber on. This helps to keep it on in case rain falls or someone graces your head in a club, or even if you are sweating.

b.   **Hats** - You can also use the old- fashioned hats or baseball caps that will of course cover your head and cover your bald spot. However, the disadvantage of this is having a job that doesn't allow hats (fedoras including) to be worn in the office. Traveling with caps on through TSA can be annoying because the moment you take it off, everyone will see your head and if someone keeps causing the metal detector to go off, it means more time for people to analyse your bald spot. Fedora hats are stylish and still cover your bald spots, but could be very hot if it's like 90 degrees outside.

c. **Bandanas** - Bandanas help to stay in style, as well hide that receding hairline, just saying.

d. **Bald Look** - Avoid up close selfies that will reveal your receding hairline unless you've shaved your head to rock a bald look with full grown beards. Cutting your hair all the way down, is less stress and worry than attempting to hide your bald spot. Everything blends in and you can rock this with full beard and mustache.

e. **Hair Pieces** - Another idea is getting realistic hair pieces or toupees. However, they can be costly as they require touch ups and refining after several weeks.

These are done by some professional barbers who have taken classes to install them. You may be required to travel to another state to get it done though, because not all hair stylists or barbers can install them properly.

f. **Durags** - Durags help you to protect your hair. They keep your waves intact, and keep your braids and dreadlocks neat while sleeping. However for this "no visible spot" tip, do-rags help to hide your bald spots while giving you style at the same time. Durags are the fastest things to use to cover your bald spots, especially when you have company arriving in a few minutes.

Durags are essential when you have no time to shave your hair for a bald look or apply hair fiber to cover your spots.

Wearing a cap/hat indoors may seem a bit too much to your guests, so I strongly advise using a durag that you can tie on your head quickly.

Taste Buds

So a few people I know have a taste buds issue that pushed them away from drinking regular water. So instead of drinking soda all the time, try these following things.

a. You can buy a bag of lemons and put slices of the lemon in your water. You can also squeeze the lemon slices in the water, satisfying your taste buds and getting you to drink more water. This helps your skin glow, aids in digestion, promotes weight loss, supports the immune system, freshens the breath and more.

b. Go for juices that are natural with no added sugars.

c. Try sparkling water, bubbly or flavored seltzer water, or carbonated water.

d. Sugar free drink mixes.

e. Make mint, cucumber or fresh fruit-flavored ice cubes to insert into your water. This will add flavor and I have heard that ice water sometimes tastes better than room temperature water.

Immune System Boosters

Immune boosters are very important to provide the necessary vitamins and important minerals to fight diseases. We shouldn't have to wait for a pandemic or to get a cold to start taking these immune system boosters. We should take these on a regular basis to protect us even before we possibly get sick.

a.   **Elderberry -** Is a fruit that is dark purple in color. It's packed with antioxidants and vitamins that help to boost your immune system. This is available in syrup form and as gummies.

b. **Blackseed Oil** - This is actually extracted oil from the seeds of Nigella sativa or fennel flower. It is mainly from Egypt and is high in antioxidants. It has a lot of health benefits that aid in boosting the immune system. This nutrient comes in a softgel capsule form and as pure cold pressed black cumin seed oil in a bottle.

c. **Sea Moss** - is also called irish moss, and is a type of seaweed that helps boost your immune system, increases metabolism, and works as an anti inflammatory. It's also an excellent source of Vitamins A, B, C & D. It gives skin support, helps in weight loss, supports sex drive, dissolves mucus and more.

d. **JackFruit** - This is an exotic or unique tropical fruit that is green in color with spikes on the outside. It has been described to taste like a mixture of mangoes, bananas, oranges and pineapples. Jackfruit is rich in folic acid, vitamin b6, magnesium, calcium, potassium and more. This fruit is also rich in Vitamin C and antioxidants which help strengthen your immune system. Jackfruit is a wonderful meat replacement for vegan dishes when the unripe flesh is cooked.

Castor Oil Magic

A lot of people overlook castor oil and its healing factors. I personally discovered castor oil can be used to slowly eliminate keloids. It was something I randomly started putting on my keloid and it reduced it dramatically. Castor oil can be used to lighten, soften and eventually eliminate keloid scars on the body. Some people crush Aspirin with a spoon and add little water to make a thick paste. They add the paste to the keloid, leave on for a few minutes till it completely dries. After washing the paste they apply castor oil. Castor oil can also be used for acne, rashes and other skin irritations. I also know it's great for skin infections & skin conditions such as boils, cystic acne and chaffing.

An Extra Push for Pregnant Women

This particular tip was shared by a friend of mine and I'm not sure why she told me. I can't give birth as a man, but I guess people love telling me the tea naturally. So I thought I'd share with you all who are pregnant or plan to be pregnant.

She was having Braxton Hicks which is a contraction but not an active labor contraction and upon visiting the doctor she had come across, a nurse that gave her a tip seeing that she was stressed with the false alarm Braxton Hicks contractions. My friend was ready to have her baby and was in pain. The nurse told her to have sex and the baby may come out sooner than expected.

They say sperm stimulates the uterus and contains things that opens it up. It helps the woman dilate and go into active labor. Do note that sex at the time of Braxton Hicks will be uncomfortable because the uterus is low.

This process is for women who have trouble giving birth and usually pass their due date. My friend spoke to the nurse that gave her this tip on Friday. She had sex that same Friday night with her husband and gave birth two days after on Sunday to a bouncing baby boy who is now putting smiles on his family's faces and pulling on his mum's wig and earrings, lol. **Please consult your doctor before trying this.**

Job

Fake It 'Till You Make It

Fake the experience till you make it. Unfortunately, we are in a generation that requires you to have 10 to 25 years of job experience and employers aren't willing to give people the opportunity to gain the experience necessary. So sometimes we have to fake it till we make it by using our friends as co-workers for verification, and if you are blessed, you can have an old manager really give you the recommendation you need and make sure they speak on things required by this new job. This is especially true for friends in the same field that can give good recommendations when they are called. We have to tweak that resume to match the requirements needed for the job.

It's a shame we have to do this, but how else can we get in the door if the owners have suddenly forgotten that someone once gave them the opportunity when they once had no experience.

An old friend of mine taught me how to walk into an establishment and follow up on my application. This shows the place that you are still interested and since you are physically there, they may interview you which is why you should dress nicely before you go there, plus it is a very good practice to make sure to take a resume. Now the real truth here is you actually have never filled out any application with them, so when they go through their system to check and they don't find your application, you have to act like "oh, I'm surprised it's not showing, I filled it out on Monday the 3rd of June at 4:14pm. Oh my god, it didn't go through? Please can you check again? My first and the last name is …." .

Usually because you're bubbly, have a personality they like, they usually will have you fill an application out again right there (al though, you are technically filling it out your first time).

Secret Siestas

Sleep break time!!! So, when you need a sleep break at work, but your work space is an office with a bunch of cameras and cubicles, I say take a quick nap in a clean environment. Sleeping in a clean bathroom never gets anyone fired or you can sleep during your break time, it's just easier.

a. Unisex bathrooms are perfect, especially the ones with seats where our sisters use to pump breast milk. Set a timer for 15 minutes and take a quick nap in the bathroom at work to get yourself together. Don't worry, if they ever put a camera in the bathroom to catch you sleeping, then you should rejoice because that's a lawsuit against them and that's retirement money, after you have been settled well depending on your starting rate or the final settlement.

b. Storage room breaks are not the most common ones, depending on the set up of your company's storage room. Sit on a strong box with your back against the door and make sure to put items (storage company supplies) on the floor in front of you. Place your back against the door so that when they open the door it will hit your back waking you (hopefully not that hard). This is when you get up halfway and scramble through the items on the floor that you placed in front of you (to act like you're arranging them) making sure you avoid eye contact so they don't see proof you were sleeping or your eyes looking sleepy, lol.

Unemployment 101

You know I have to say America did a fine job with the idea of unemployment for those who lost their jobs. There are so many countries that don't have this and I know it would be beneficial for them. This really does help people keep their sanity while searching for opportunities to get back on their feet.

We do find ourselves in situations where the job is toxic and you just can't walk out or you won't be covered by unemployment. Do you need unemployment but you are tired of your toxic job? Always remember never to quit a job unless you were sexually harassed or certain other intense situations occurred.

As for other situations, you have to let them let you go (terminate you) so you can get unemployment. If they discuss something, you should write responses through email, including appropriate people from the conflict, even including the person in your emails who usually accepts or declines unemployment when you apply. Remember emails protect you when you need to fight the job for your unemployment. Save your receipts from emails, to your performances, and more. If you were laid off, then it's an easier process to get your unemployment and it's pretty much automatic.

Keep in mind that it's really hard to get in contact with unemployment offices, so it's better to call them early in the morning when they open. Also, messaging them on their official twitter through the dm works.

They have an automated response through the twitter dm that schedules a call with you within 2-3 business days. I would suggest doing the application for unemployment online on their websites, rather than trying to call to get it done. When you also sign up for direct deposit, your payments come in quicker.

Note - Make sure the online unemployment application you fill out is on the official website and that you get email receipts or text receipts after filling out the application. During the 2020 pandemic, there were fake websites which had what looked like the official unemployment application and these websites were designed to steal your information and also to get your payments.

The tea that got delivered to my doorstep is that when you fill out these applications on these fake sites, the person who made this fraudulent website takes all your info and fills it out the real application on the official website with all your info, replacing your direct deposit info with theirs, then collects your money on your behalf.

Put It In Writing

Do you have a shady job? Then everything or most things should be in writing. When you communicate, especially through emails, you are able to save these as receipts (receipts meaning proof of communications, etc). Even if the supervisor is beside you and you need to speak to her about something troubling your mind that you felt was wrong, put it in writing.

 If the supervisor, however, does have a verbal communication with you, you can still go back to your desk after like an hour and send an email that says something like "thank you so much for listening to my concerns about my co-worker who has been unprofessional to me during our meetings. I hope proper actions will be taken ….". Always print or email yourself your receipts to a personal email address, because your work email can be deleted by the company and if you're terminated you may not get access to it after that moment. Always remember that things said verbally can not be proven, so try to email things more so you have necessary proof and save yourself with the email tracking records.

This really helps when you need to fight a case for unemployment or prove any kind of case that may ask for proof.

Questionable Contracts

We all need to be very comfortable with reading contracts given to us. If you don't understand the contract, you can get a trustworthy friend to read over it with you. If you can get a lawyer to go through it, then do so. Don't be afraid to ask for a few more minutes to read it through before signing. Most importantly, don't be afraid to negotiate some part of the contracts, regardless of who it is with.

Sometimes receiving contracts that will get you millions, makes you want to sign immediately before they change their minds. But it's more important to ask questions and change things if needed because you don't want to sign today and regret later when you are stuck working for them till your age 65 according to what you signed because you didn't read or negotiate. The worst thing is signing a contract and later finding out that you don't even own your name or anything you have written or produced and all of it is owned by the company. Understand NDAs that you sign as well, thoroughly, so as not to get yourself in big trouble.

Money

Extra Money

There is never enough money. This is for those of us who are just not comfortable being naked in front of the camera or on onlyfans. Not all of us want to get paid to flirt with strangers (yes, that is a thing. If you're interested, just google "Get paid to flirt with Men Online" and you will stumble across so many companies that will pay you to just text random strangers. All you have to do is flirt.) Kudos to the only-fans individuals making their coins. Oh, and if you want to be a dominatrix on the side (a dominatrix is someone who inflicts pain on someone usually a partner or client who finds the pain to be sexually satisfying. The person enjoying the pain can be slapped, whipped or beaten with a paddle stick), I heard they make good money. Their clients pay very well to be humiliated and abused.

So, for the rest of us who can't do the above, we can do the following.

a. **Focus Groups & Opinion Research Studies** - This is sitting with a group of people discussing items or products a company just introduced and they are paying you for your opinion whether good or bad. I have gone to one about potato chips, was there for one hour, and was paid $250 for my opinion.

b. **Sleep Studies** - Some sleep studies, usually health related, may require you to sleep in for a couple of days and they will watch you on their monitors to see your sleep pattern, depending on the case they are working. Keep in mind they may ask you to take pills, again depending on what they are observing you for. These pay a lot, I just never tried these studies as I do not feel comfortable putting pills in my mouth.

c. **Secret Shopper** - Secret shopping is another activity to make money. This is when the company pays you to go to their store and act like you're shopping. They want you to report back to them concerning your shopping experience, whether it was good or bad. Most times, only 30 minutes of your time is required and they can pay from $100 to maybe $300 dependent upon the task or what they will ask you to do specifically in the store.

To find all three of these money making

activities, you can google them. For example, search for "focus groups in New York". Don't forget they will ask you screening questions/surveys to see if you qualify for the study. So if you don't drink beer and the study is on beer, they will know based on the questions they ask unless you are a good liar, but that's none of my business.

Invest

Investment provides the highest potential returns. It's very easy to invest and this helps to save for retirement. This helps to grow your wealth and also is a great way to grow your savings over time. You can start with investments apps or you can even attend online classes to learn. Once you start investing you can reduce the risk of losing investment money by investing in many companies instead of only one company. You learn a lot about investing this way, especially when you invest in your favorite companies and make money while doing so.

Know the Right Payment Services

So, there are a ton of payment services out there, but not all are helpful to get your money back especially when you've made payments to the wrong person or been a victim of a fraudulent business deal.

I personally only use Cash App or Venmo when I'm paying for something that's already in my hands and I double check the name to be sure before clicking send. I do not usually use these for example, when it's an expected service that's not going to be rendered much later in the month. Once you send money through Cash App and Venmo, it is gone and can't be returned.

Let me tell you all a story. There was a time I paid for a pop-up shop space and I paid a month in advance. The day came for the event and I arrived to come set up. I was first, shown the coat check to set up my t-shirts, books and other items from my boutique. I didn't even move an inch and I immediately asked for the person I had paid money to.

Not only were they telling me to set up in a coat check section, but also to set up in that same place with a food vendor who seemed comfortable setting up her cookies and cakes in that space. I was trying to understand why she would want us to set up in that space. I truly believe that wasn't a good representation of one's brand to be seen setting up in a coat rack space. There were times people reached to grab

84

for the snacks and thought the food was free because again it was in the coat check section. So, she ended up giving the snacks free to people in frustration as she couldn't take them back home she said. Eventually, the person I had paid my money to arrived, but he gave me a small table and placed it in the dark near a stage where performances were taking place, with people standing close to the table. If I had accepted it, anyone could have stolen my merchandise in the dark and as they would be standing over me, there is no way anyone would notice a table in that space. I told him I would not accept it and I wanted a refund. He agreed, but it was a different story when I got home. I told Venmo what happened, thinking they would help me out. Even when I showed proof of our email exchanges that showed the agreement of my refund, Venmo basically told me there is nothing they could do. So I called Chase Bank to get my money back, showing all the proof needed and finally, Chase got my money back. Venmo was expecting me to pay the money back that Chase took, and obviously I'm not going to do that, so I just took it as I'm blocked.

I always suggest using PayPal, especially when you click the buyer protection program for services. That way, if you pay good money for something of value and in return the service was a 99 cent value, you can get your money back by calling PayPal as long as you sent the money through the buyer protection option for services.

The buyer protection program is offered by

PayPal. It helps protect buyers from fraud especially when the item you received is not what was shown or the item never arrived.This helps to get your money back from the seller.

Used But New Money

I didn't know that you could sell your used clothes to make money until I heard it on the radio. So selling clothes to consignment shops is a way to make money, for sure. However, keep in mind that they don't take everything and the clothes they may take depends upon the season, and the age/wear of the clothing.

They will buy jeans, t-shirts, halloween costumes, dresses, wedding gowns and more. It's important to bring the clothes very clean and in great condition to be able to get as much money as possible from each item. Selling our used clothes, aside from getting money, helps to get rid of the clothes taking space in our closets.

Also these shops do sell very unique items in their stores, so after you drop off your clothes to sell, I do recommend walking around to check out unique finds you can purchase depending on your taste or comfort.

Sexual

Bagsexual

In the midst of giving a few beneficial tips and amazing tricks, I just have to spill the tea. Sometimes I don't know what it is, but the tea always gets delivered to my doorstep. So I thought I would share this tea with sugar and not sea salt. Bagsexual means a man who often claims to be straight but is willing do anything or certain things with other males for money, career upgrades or a better social status. Bagsexual also means gay for pay.

Rub his head, stroke his ego, be desperate and offer money, they say for a man who is bagsexual, and they will fall right into the trap. Society today says everyone has a price.

a.   **The Types** - The Social media male models, fitness trainers, your local weed man and upcoming music artists are a few examples of guys who can be bagsexual and sometimes have a price, especially when you slide in DMs or text them. Believe it or not, they some times have a wealthy man who is sponsoring their trips, education, careers and even harder to believe taking care of their wives and kids.

b.   **OnlyFans** - The OnlyFans website we think we know is not just an online content sharing platform for people who have fans. The content creators have made pages on OnlyFans that have become a gateway passage for other things. They get requests for custom videos where they show their butt to male fans, or even requests to show their feet. They even sell worn and cum stained underwear to customers and they use toys (dildos etc) in the videos for their paying male customers. They even charge for FaceTime shows where they do whatever the male paying customers ask them to do. Lastly, depending on how much you are willing to spend, you could meet them in person for a full course meal.

c. **Deep Divers** - We often know of these guys that intentionally join gay websites just for the cash. They know guys will rush them with the dollars, so they go straight to the well and they do make loads of cash. Going in with no emotional attachments, they offer massages and more, depending on how much you are willing to spend.

Your tax returns are their pleasures, your stimulus checks are their needs and your approved grant money is their life source. Everyone has got to make a living and I'm not here to judge.

I'm just here letting y'all know what's going on, that's all. Once they start getting money from all corners, it's hard to stop and they always come back for more.

Just Hooking Up

Unsure Hookups - There comes a time in one's life when someone wants to release some tension. We just want to hook up. So, if you are inviting the person over to your place and you are unsure if they are crazy or not, it's always okay to try this.

a. For example, if your building has security at the front desk, don't be afraid to use it to your advantage by saying to the person through text that "oh, the police officer or security guard will let you in, but I'm not sure who is on duty." This will have him or her on his or her toes to not try any BS. It puts them on alert and if they are not sincere, usually they find an immediate excuse and cancel.

b. Also, you can say a neighbor is a police officer, he or she will be on edge and wouldn't want any BSing.

c. You can also say "Yes, I stay alone, but my uncle is in town helping the police force with a joint task. He is staying with me and he has the keys." This helps just in case when they arrive the person is not attractive to you and they decide to stay on their own terms. So, if they are not cute when they walk in, you can easily say, "Oh damn, my uncle is almost here." However, if they are cute and you feel safe with them, just go ahead and tell them you told your uncle to call you before he leaves his job and go ahead and have some fun.

d. The safe way is the way to be in control.

Meeting outside, talking over the phone first and FaceTiming just helps to avoid catfish and more. Sometimes you can lie that your friend is outside in their car waiting for you guys to hook up and finish (this keeps a crazy person from carrying out their crazy plans as they do not like too many eyes on them).

e. Retract messages on WhatsApp, and Insta gram, for people you are just not sure of yet and may say stuff that you may need to delete after.

f. People who ask for a whole photo album on a hook up site are red flags! Two photos are fine. All these "I want body pics", "I need a full photo", "what's your Instagram" messages are a waste of time. Ain't nobody got time for that.

g. Use fake numbers to chat, as people search your number and find you on Facebook/IG using your number. I guess not everyone understands no strings attached. So, download the Text Apps (TextNow, TextFree & TextPlus to name a few) to chat or call.

h. Afraid of someone exposing your nudes is understandable. If you're at their house, check for camera lights and laptops. Don't ever take a full nude with your face. Even when you send ass pics, try to not to send ass and face pics so close during the messages. You're better off hosting, as they say, than traveling. Try sending photos through an app that lets the photos disappear after they click the photo once.

X-rated Tips

Here are sexual tips to ensure actual safety. The tea that was delivered to my doorstep taught me on some of these points below. I also have had personal experiences with one or two of these points as well.

a.   **Don't Get Drugged** - First we were worried about our drinks being spiked now we have to worry about something else. For those of us that use lube to have sex or use lube to be penetrated, I have some tea for you. The tea is it's better to bring or use your own lube. Apparently, some people insert drugs (GHB and GBL) into the lube.

This allows the mixture to be injected anally,

causing the mixture to be absorbed more quickly into the bloodstream which results in an immediate and intense effect. This leaves the victim overdosed to be taken advantage of. The drugger could take your naked photos, rape you or even invite friends to join him in raping you. Please be careful.

b. **Guide Your Condoms** - You have to make sure the person you are having sex with actually puts the condom on completely. Some people are on a mission to purposely pass things on to others, or some people want to have raw sex even though you already said no. You have to use your hand to inspect the penis that will be penetrating with the condom on using your hand to guide it in while rubbing it and checking if the condom is on. You will be surprised how many people remove the condoms the moment you turn your face away and they are about to go in you. Some even cut the top of the condom to make it seem like the condom ripped while you were having sex.

c. **Dispose Properly** – It's important to throw your condoms away yourself by wrapping it up in a toilet paper and not putting down the toilet.

However, the reason I mentioned throwing away your condoms yourself is good is because some women may have other plans with your sperm, especially if they want to be attached to you for life and financially. They could easily use a turkey baster to

103

suck the contents (sperm) in the condom to artificially inseminate themselves without your knowledge to get pregnant.

d. **Pep** - For some reason, if you just happen to find yourself having sex raw because you were drunk, drugged or the guy or girl was super hot and you decided to go raw because there were no condoms available, I have a 72 hour solution. The word is PEP (post - exposure prophylaxis). Go to your nearest clinics or hospitals to get it within 72 hours if you feel you may have been exposed to HIV. This however will be taken for 28 days. Also there are some government funded and local free medical clinics that can give you Pep for free. These clinics have tons of free condoms and lube also, if needed. For more info contact your doctor as I am not a medical professional, however this totally saved my life.

e. **Prep** - Pre-exposure prophylaxis helps to prevent the risk of getting HIV. This has to be taken consistently so if you do have a slip up, you sort of are protected. However, this should be used along with condoms. You can get more info from your doctors. Also, there are some government funded and local free medical clinics that can give you Prep for free. For more info, contact your doctor as I am not a licensed medical professional.

f. **Poppers** - This is a liquid drug that helps a person to feel relaxed mentally and physically with an increased sexual arousal. This drug helps to make anal sex so much easier by relaxing the anal muscles and makes it less painful especially if your partner is big or you are just not used to anal sex. It also aids in enhanced orgasm.

NOTE - Use poppers at your own risk. They have side effects that affect blood pressure, may give you a headache and more. Make sure you do more research and read more on these and use at your own risk. Check if your city allows them as I have heard some places have them banned. To get them into the country, sometimes they are labelled as nail polish removers. They can be found at your local sex store or online.

g. Always remember condoms have expiration

dates on them (a lot of people don't know this) and oral condoms are not for anal sex or vaginal sex.

h. Be careful of people that ask if you are "Gen" and if you "Party". These questions are usually asked in gay apps. When someone "asks are you gen?" it means are you generous with money. What they are truly asking is if you are generous enough to give them money, usually for sexual favors. Most of the times the people who ask these questions are going through financial difficulties and are willing to do anything sexual as long as you are generous. Now if someone asks "do you party?", it means do you do drugs and the most common one is called "Tina" or "T" which is crystal meth.

Depending on the form, it can be sniffed, swallowed, injected and it is white in color. It comes in different forms such as powder, tablets and crystals. Usually people that use this drug get an intense high and have a high sexual drive while they are high. Most of the times they have no idea if the person they are having sex with, or about to have sex with, has a condom on or not because they are way to high to even notice or care. It gets them super high and the important thing at the moment is to have sex. The tina often has them acting confused and sometimes even aggressive. A number of people on the apps seem to party a lot and are seeking generous men.

Stay Ready

This will only apply to those who enjoy the pleasure of anal sex and find ways to avoid embarrassments when they have sexual relations. There is the typical way of douching which includes using a douche bulb filled with water or another safe solution which is inserted into your rectum to flush out any possible poop. However, this is not for everyone and it is also not the safest route, especially when done too often or excessively. It's always best to consult your doctor before using this method.

Aside from douching, there is a fiber supplement pill that can provide the same cleanliness results as douching. One pill that is popular right now is "Pure for Men" which is a fiber capsule that contains chia, flaxseed and psyllium husk. Pure for Men has instructions on the daily usage and emphasizes drinking a lot of water. Keep in mind what you eat and the timing of your movements. It is expected to be taken daily to work well and for your body to adjust to it.

For more info check the Pure for Men website. Also check with your doctor to make sure you can use this along with any other thing you may be using already. Lastly, have fun!

Social & Everyday Life Activities

Drinking 101

We all think we know how to handle ourselves or know how we act or react, but when we start gulping shots, then we become someone else.

a. **Big Meal** - Eating before drinking allows a higher tolerance for alcohol. Eating a big meal before drinking keeps you more sober.

b. **Beware** – Be careful who you drink around. People that offer to go in the uber with the person who is drunk are not always good people. They can ride that uber with you, take you straight to bed and you wake up with them beside you. They probably would have already have taken advantage of you by morning time.

c. **Bathroom Restrictions** - Only let someone you trust in the bathroom with you when you're drunk. I have seen situations when perverts will follow someone into the bathroom and act like they are helping but really are taking a peek at the drunk person's private parts.

They can even take pictures of your private parts while you're drunk. Even if they offer to hold your phone, they could be scrolling through to send your nudes to themselves and delete traces. How do I know this? I always get the tea delivered to my doorstep.

d. **Reminders** - Never turn your back on your

drink or walk away from your drink. Also, never let a stranger bring a drink over to you randomly. You may have heard this, but this is a reminder.

Good Gifts 101

a.   **Gift Cards** - Birthday cards with gift cards and wine bottles with birthday cards save the day! This is an easy way out when you don't have time to dig through the mall. When you give them gift cards, they can go out and buy what they want, or use it to see a movie, or even pay for dinner.

b. **Customized Pieces** - Customized items are unique presents and most people love unique items. You can have a jacket customized, or even a bag customized with the person's name or initials, depending on their style.

c. **Stocks** - Buy stocks for your kids, nephews,

and nieces. If they are kids under legal age, you can set up an account for them which you can manage until they are of age. Trust me, this will be appreciated when they are of age: when they are off to college or when they want to rent their first apartment. It could be helpful even if they want to start a business at a young age.

Luggage Drama

a. **Luggage Digital Weight** - To avoid over-weight items at the airport, its best to buy a digital weight scale from your nearest store to be prepared. That way you can remove items to adjust to the allowed baggage weight. My fellow Nigerians need this item for sure. It should be included as a birthday gift to someone who travels a lot with overweight bags.

b. **Roll Your Clothes** - Rolling your clothes, rather than folding them, saves you a lot of space so you can actually include more items in the luggage.

c. **The Right Luggage** - If you are the type that packs a lot, make sure to buy the right luggage that actually has a lot of space inside. What is the use of fancy luggage that doesn't have any space? This will only have you walking through the airport with 8 bags.

Ottomans

Ottomans are key. They have multiple functions within an apartment. This is especially true in small spaces like studio apartments. You can save all your precious junk in there, and still be neat and tidy. They can also be used as coffee tables and are great for foot rests. They are fashionable as well, and can be chosen to match the rest of your decor by just getting the right design, size and/or color.

Refreshing Escapes

Perfect Phone Escape Routes -

a. If you are on FaceTime when it is refreshing or loses signal, that is the perfect time to hang up on that annoying guy or girl, friend or family member who doesn't schedule a FaceTime with you.

b. Sometimes it's better to hang up and switch off the phone on your annoying noisy friend who wants gossip on your relationship. Then text them later saying, "Sorry, my phone died and I just found the charger".

c. You can always say Mum is calling or texting you about an emergency, etc.

d. Don't feel like talking? Let it ring and call the person back at 1am when obviously they will be asleep and you know for sure they will be asleep. Just simply text them around 1am or 2am saying " hey girl, hey my bad, I just woke up, I'll call you tomorrow". This also works for people who text you and are annoying juts; ignore the text and reply much later. You can text them back at a late hour (1, 2 or 3am for example) when they are already sleeping; by doing this it will assure you that they won't reply immediately because they are sleeping and you can also feel assured that you did at least respond.

e. Now you have some annoying people who claim there is an emergency and they are texting and calling you, but they have a history of their emergencies just being gossip. So for these people, honestly, if it's an emergency they should call 911 point blank period!. There's no law that says you have to answer your phone.

f. When the person receives a call on the other line and switches over. You can easily text them while they are speaking to say "hey girl let me call you back real quick".

Negative Escape Routes -

We all may have been in situations where people invite you to places and you don't really fancy their friends or people they hang out with. This is usually why most people ask, "Who will be there?"

a. Honestly, you can decline the offer from the beginning, because if it requires fake smiling then you probably shouldn't go. Say something else is planned for the day. A simple hello to you from someone who caused you pain can set you off unexpectedly, so it's better to not even go.

b. If you find yourself seated at a table with someone you no longer are interested in or are not friends with anymore, and you really don't want to go to jail for beating up this fellow, it's better to just straight get up from the table and walk out. You can do this or say you need to use the restroom and exit (just make sure your items are paid for before leaving but usually I advise to get only water when you know you are about to exit).

This is way better than causing a scene at a restaurant or going to jail for fighting.

c. We all have friends who want you to speak to the other friend you had a falling out with. People don't understand things until it's done to them, so if you are invited somewhere and you know for a fact the person you don't want to see is going be there, just simply tell them you can't be in the same space with the person anywhere or ever at all, especially if you are mentally not ready. Hopefully the person will understand and it's not their wedding day where they will be very upset if you don't attend .

Very Questionable Energies

I am learning to keep so many things to myself, especially great news or potentially big deals. Sometimes peoples' energy can literally destroy that opportunity or take away that big deal because their energy is wrapped with unintentional jealousy which they themselves are potentially unaware of. Not everyone is happy for you, sometimes they usually start with the "you have changed" statement and then they stop inviting you to places. Sometimes "friends" can be mad at you because you are doing better than them or because you decided to better yourself and they didn't. Those are not your friends; your friends will celebrate with you no matter what.

Know the energy around you and observe the

"fun shade" constantly thrown at you.

Remember energy doesn't lie.

Washroom Diaries

For this part of the book I'm certainly not telling you how to wash your bathroom or how to wash your toilet or how to wash your mirror. I'm pointing at the main embarrassing thing.

Smelly Poop - When you are stuck in someone's bathroom and there's no air freshener.

a. Just squeeze hand soap from the sink in the toilet before you poop, squeeze it on your poop and flush to avoid embarrassing smells at someone's house.

b. If worse comes to worse and they just don't have air fresheners or hand soap that's squeezable, just see if they have bleach and pour it in the toilet. The smell of bleach will surely overpower the poopy smell. Yup, your welcome.

c. Reach in their cabinet and spray their cologne. Be mindful, they may curse you out for touching things in their cabinet, but if they are your close friends and family, and you're at a house party, this is necessary to avoid embarrassment, especially if people are waiting at the door.

d. **Toilet Spray** - This is usually a small spray bottle that has different scents. It's a pocket size that makes it easy to take with you. You are supposed to spray it into the toilet, over the toilet water, before you sit down to do your thing. You could spray the toilet right after you flush as well to really make sure it eliminates any smell, but usually the first spray before you sit on the toilet is enough.

You Just Never Know

You just never know what people are going through privately. So, in your spare time, please check on your friends, family members, co-workers, etc. A friendly text, phone call, social media dm or a visit to their home is fine. Suicide rates are still high. It's heartbreaking in general, but hurts even more when it's someone you thought was good because you see them posting on Facebook, Twitter, TikTok or Instagram. You just never know what people are going through, regardless of whether they seem happy to you.

Ripped Pants

Some of us have big thighs which cause stress on the seams when rubbed together. Our jeans/pants just rip in the middle of the inseam. We may not be close to a store to change our pants, sometimes we may not even have the immediate funds for new pants, so we have to wait to shop.

a.   Throw a long sweater on to cover it depending on the weather and where you are.

b.   Tie your outer shirt/sweater around your waist for a fashion statement, while still covering the hole. The sleeves when tied fall to the front and will dangle in the middle area of your waist, covering the rip or tear in the pants. The back area is spread wide when tied, so it covers the back area of your pants if your pants ripped at the back.

c. You can buy a mini sewing case that has the needle, thread and small scissors. Throw it in your purse, leave it in your car, leave it at your office. You can sew your pants quickly in the bathroom or in the car.

Opening Stubborn Lids

Hopefully you are somewhere that has these items that can aid to open stubborn jars that have pickles and other things you salivate to eat quickly.

a. **Rubber Band** - Find a tight fitting rubberband (a single thick rubber band or 2 maybe 3 rubber band pieces) and place it on the lid. Once it's on the lid, grab the lid with your entire palms and turn firmly to open.

b. **Gloves** - A kitchen glove or disposable glove can be worn and then you can grab the lid with your entire palm. Once you grab the lid firmly with your entire palm, you can turn firmly to open.

Know Your Circle Test

There are ways to tell if someone is trustworthy within an office or group of friends. This works way better when you tell only one person. Tell the person, for example, you have an upcoming project with a huge celeb or huge department.

Tell the person not to tell anyone and see if it finds its way back to you. There may be someone texting you or calling you starting with "hey I heard".

Sometimes you have to also test physically by leaving certain items on the table to see if someone is trustworthy to bring to your house again. The old trick is leaving a few dollars that you are okay losing.

You basically leave a few dollars on the table and see if it goes missing. I wouldn't necessarily try this with a friend as it seems disrespectful and the person shouldn't be considered a friend if you can't trust them from the beginning .

Memorizing Important Numbers

This may seem silly to some readers, however, I feel it's very important. People get arrested for crimes and people also get arrested wrongfully. It would be annoying and frustrating to be locked up for something you consider not valid enough to be handcuffed and taken to the police station or jail. You could be arrested for defending yourself against someone who attacked you first, and a partner or family member could lie that you hit them when they dial 911. When these police officers arrest you there is not enough time to go through your phone to call anyone. Even when you get to the station, they take your belongings away from you. They do allow you to make a call from the pay phone, however you won't be allowed to check your phone. So this is why it's necessary to memorize important people's phone numbers so you can call your partner, friend or family member to come get you out. It's also important to remember phone numbers if you are stranded somewhere and your phone may have died, then you can ask to use a strangers phone. But if you don't remember any numbers, then you are screwed. It's very important to memorize people's numbers who are reliable and who usually pick up their phone.

Manufacturing Info

This information is mostly for those looking to get into clothing businesses. This particular tip is very hard to come by, but I thought I should share this just in case someone may get lucky. On some popular brands they may leave some information for you by mistake. Check the inside of the item, T-shirts for example, and check the care instructions label. When you do this you just may come across manufacturing information the manufacturing company forgot to remove or added by mistake.

I once bought an item from a popular brand and I found the manufacturing tag once. I immediately called the manufacturing company to ask questions and more. Keep in mind most of these manufacturing companies will require you to have a large minimum amount to order from them or for them to begin production. I hope you are able to come across a manufacturing label from a brand you admire and then can also produce a high quality clothing line. It's very rare that people or these popular brands share these types of information, even when you go to their physical or online workshops. Good luck on your journey!

Thank you so much for being open to reading this book. I hope you find the information in this book helpful.

You can view more of my work on my website at www.BiodunAbudu.com

Feel free to write me at info@biodunabudu.com

Acknowledgments

A special thanks to the following people:

Katherine Knott
(Genesis Design and Editing LLC)

Henry Jimenez

Christel Rodriguez

You all made this book possible!

ABOUT THE AUTHOR

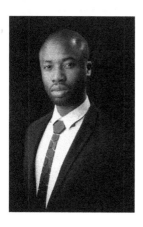

Biodun Abudu was born in Rhode Island, but comes from a Nigerian background. He wrote his first title, "Tales of My Skin", based on a true life story in 2011. He then released his second title "Stolen Sanity", in 2019, which is also based on a true life story. His third book, "Forbidden Scriptures", was released in 2020. When he is not writing, he works as an artist. In 2011, he graduated with an A.S. degree in Fashion Design, and a B.A. in Merchandising Management with an emphasis on Fashion Merchandising. He currently resides in New York City.

Email : info@biodunabudu.com

Website : www.BiodunAbudu.com

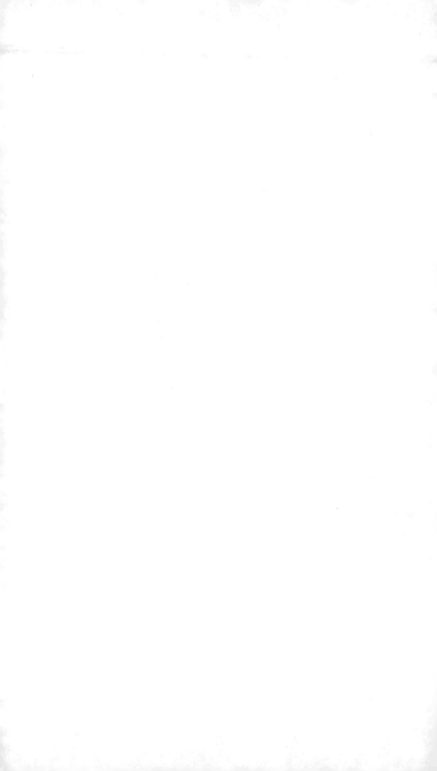

www.ingramcontent.com/pod-product-compliance
Lightning Source LLC
Chambersburg PA
CBHW071131050326
40690CB00008B/1428